R. U. LIVEN-WELL

Muscle Building Routine

Fundamentals to adding lean muscle fast

First edition

This book was professionally typeset on Reedsy.
Find out more at reedsy.com

"Some people want it to happen, some wish
it would happen, others make it happen."

Michael Jordan

Contents

1

Introduction

Welcome to the *Introductory Series: How to Develop a Muscle Building Routine the Fundamentals of Building Lean Muscle FAST,* where we will discuss the fundamentals of establishing and developing a routine to building lean muscle fast. The topics discussed in this book will be relevant whether you are just starting your fitness journey, an intermediate gym enthusiast or a pure gym rat looking to brush up on your knowledge. This is a topic that gets me excited just thinking about it and I can't wait to support your journey. Throughout my journey of 10+ years, i am looking forward to sharing some tricks of the trade using my personal experience of trial-and-error to learn the most effective and efficient way to improve overall health, fitness and physique.

When it comes to building muscle, this can be achieved in multiple ways with different types of training. The two most discussed are either strength training or hypertrophy training. Both methods will allow you to achieve muscle growth as well as strength gain. But each has a primary goal that differs. Let's take moment to look at the two.

Hypertrophy training has a primary goal of increasing muscle size and mass with a secondary benefit of getting stronger.

Strength training has a primary goal of gaining overall strength with a secondary benefit of gaining muscle as a secondary benefit.

This is not to say that one training method is better than the other. They are both forms of resistance training that will essentially help you achieve varying levels of the same benefits. I find it best to cycle through different training methods periodically as your body will adapt and plateau casing the level of gains to level off. For the sake of this book, we will be focusing on Hypertrophy training. Don't worry, we will not get overly scientific and I will keep it as simple as possible.

First, I would like to start off by addressing a couple of anticipated questions that may have come to mind.

Who is this book for?

This book is perfect for men and women of all ages that are seeking to gain a baseline fundamental knowledge with a drive and aspiration of improving their overall health, fitness and physique. It doesn't matter if you are trying to bulk up or just simply trying to improve your overall physique, you'll be able to find something that is easily applicable and relevant to your current and or new routines.

What to expect?

Anticipate gaining a better knowledge of what you can easily incorporate into your existing routines or develop a new routine. Keep in mind that everyone is different in the way that they react to different levels of stresses throughout the fitness journey due to age, gender, genetic background, time available, access to equipment, etc. Therefore, everyone's level of development and results will vary. This book is meant to be used as a guide to determine what works best for you.

Why should I read this book?

If you are currently reading this book, I do not have to share that the benefits of physical exercise has endless rewards that not only apply to your physical appearance but across life in general such as overall improved health, increased strength, better mobility, potential decreased risk of injury and chronic disease, you get to eat more calories, etc. Not to mention that you will finally get the attention of your secret crush next time you run into them… The goal of this book is to help you achieve your personal goals quickly.

With all this said, I am inspired and motivated to help guide you along the way. Let's dive in!

2

Establishing a Routine

L et's start off with a couple of fundamentals to get oriented as you setup or adjust your routine. Keep in mind that there are multiple factors to consider, life events and schedules change taking into account work, family, social life, etc. Unless your schedule is set and doesn't change, it can be like trying to hit multiple moving targets at the same time. Therefore, the key here is to be resilient and adaptable. It is OK If your kids must stay home sick, your boss asks for you to come in early for that project you have been working on, you have a night out with friends and sleep in, etc. You will be OK. You may just need to shift things around to accommodate and work out in the morning, or during your lunch break, after the kids go down to sleep or skip a day getting back on track the following day. If you have the desire, you will find a way. Let's looks at a couple of additional items to keep in mind.

Timing

It doesn't matter when you start your routine – morning, afternoon or nighttime. So long as you get your time in. This can be flexible from day to day or month to month. The main thing is that you adequately plan your scheduling. It makes things a lot easier to have a consistent schedule, i.e. workout every morning or before lunch, but is not necessary. The key part here is to ensure that you are planning well in advance to allow ample time to fuel up with a meal well in advance and to stay hydrated. If you plan to work out at night, make sure you have ample time to relax before going to sleep as this wind down process can take a while. Also try and get around 24 hours in between workout sessions to allow you body to recover. For example, if you work out at night and then first thing in the morning, yes this is technically the next day, but you may not be fully recovered hindering your results. This is a general guideline and not mandatory but try to stay closer to the 24-hour mark.

Warm Up

It is also a very beneficial to perform a light warm up prior to getting started through some light cardio, stretching, foam rolling, etc. The benefit of a warm-up acts as a primer to get your body in the ideal state physically as it will help to elevate your body temperature to increase the blood flow. This time will also allow you to prep mentally as you embrace the new challenges ahead of you. A warm up routine doesn't have to be a long elaborate process. Just enough to loosen your body up, get a light sweat going and prevent injury.

As you progress into more complex and difficult movements, it is also best to get in adequate warm up sets prior to jumping into your working weight. To do this is very simple, start as low as possible and work your way up. For example, if doing a movement that requires a barbell, start with just the barbell working with perfect form focusing on the intended muscle group being worked. If using dumbbells, start as light as possible and do the same. As you become more comfortable with the more complex movements, you can decrease the amount of warm up sets and increase the warm up weight. As you become comfortable a good warm up would be to perform 1-3 sets at between 35% to 75% of your target weight.

Form

I would be remiss if we didn't state an obvious but one of the most overlooked topics – Form. It is crucial to ensure we keep our egos in check making sure we concentrate on keeping the best form possible. This means that if we need to lighten the load and take off a plate (or two) to ensure that we are moving in as perfect form as possible, do it. This will help with injury prevention as well as ensuring that the primary muscle group you intend to work, is getting worked. Most movements activate multiple muscle groups, but we usually have a primary muscle group we intend to work. As you fatigue, it is inevitable for other muscles to kick in but we want to delay and or prevent as much as possible. Keep a straight spine with controlled movements.

Rep Range

The target number of reps to be used per each set is called your rep range. Depending on the end goal – muscle gain, strength gain, weight loss, endurance training, etc. – the rep range will vary. For our goal in establishing a muscle gaining program through hypertrophy, the rep range that should be used is between 8-12 reps. This is a good working range to work with that will allow adequate volume. The range will also let you know if you are lifting too much or not enough weight. If you start hitting 12 reps with more in the tank, time to go up in weight. If you struggle to get 8 reps in, might be time to lower the weight. Main thing, ensure you keep good form throughout all reps.

Load

The workload or load refers to the weight x volume, i.e. 185 lbs for 8 reps = 1,480 lbs load. We want to ensure that we are (1) getting enough volume to force your muscles to grow as well as (2) the working weight is progressively increasing throughout the program. The key here is to know your limits. A good way to do this is by ensuring that you know how many more reps you can do before failure and if the weight is allowing you to hold good form. Yes, it can be appealing to slam plate after plate onto the barbell or let the heavy dumb bells slam on the ground after a set on the bench, hoping your gym crush sees you, but this is also how the injuries pop up. Check the ego and make sure you know your limits.

Progressive Overload

Now that you know how much weight to use for each movement as a baseline, we need to ensure that we are pushing the limits in a way to ensure we are not exposing ourselves to injury. Progressive overload is a technique used to continuously improve or increase the workload. This can be done many ways. To keep it simple, just as add more weight or add more reps, while holding good form. With the continued increasing workload, you will be placing more stress on your body forcing it to grow. Measure the total volume of the workload each session to ensure you are progressively overloading for growth.

An example of this would be as follows:

Week 1 – Flat Bench with Barbell

3 (sets) x 8 (reps) x 185 lb (load) = 4,440 lbs (total workload)

Week 2 – Flat Bench with Barbell
   3 (sets) x 9 (reps) x 185 lb (load) = 4,995 lbs (total workload)
   or
   3 (sets) x 8 (reps) x 190 lb (load) = 4,560 lb (total workload)

In the example above, simply by adding 1 more rep or an additional 5 lbs (2 x 2.5 lb plates), you are increasing your total workload / volume by either 555 lbs or 120 lbs respectively. By following this week in and week out your muscles will be forced to grow. Keep in mind that you may only be able to do an extra rep on the first set and the same number of reps on the following sets. That's OK as well. As long as we are progressing and holding good form.

Time Under Tension

Time under tension simply refers to the duration that your muscles are under tension or being worked. Time under tension is made up of two parts – a concentric and an eccentric phase. A concentric movement is when you are contracted your muscle or shortening the muscle. This can also be referred to as the *positive* portion of the movement. The second phase is the eccentric movements which is the opposite – the lengthening of the muscle or referred to as the *negative* portion of the movement. Both phases play a key role in maximize your growth.

Nearly every exercise will have both a concentric and an eccentric movement which will help in activating multiple types of muscle fibers. For muscle gaining goals, it is important to focus on both movements with intention. A good rule of thumb would be to have a quicker concentric movement with a slight pause focusing on contracting the muscle at the top with a slow eccentric movement (around 3 seconds) lengthening the muscle. Note that this will be more difficult and will be absolutely draining, so go a bit lighter at first.

3

Nutrition

One of the biggest drivers and contributors to gaining muscle comes down to nutrition and the overall number of calories you are taking in. Along with total calorie count, you also want to concentrate on the quality of calories as well. For the sake of making overall muscular gains, you need to be in a what is called a *caloric surplus*, which is exactly what is sounds like. You need to intake more calories than you are burning throughout the day from things such as daily activities, exercise, sleeping, etc. This is opposed to when you are seeking to lose weight or entering a cutting phase whereas you need to be in a caloric deficit, i.e. taking in less calories than you are burning throughout the day. With this said, let's break this down into two sections – total calorie count and Macro counts.

When trying to identify how many calories you need to gain muscle, you will find many different complex calculations, methods, theories, etc. Depending on how far along your fitness journey you are, you can calculate a number of different ways. As this is an introductory series, we will do our best to make this as easy as possible and focus on two items here – Your BMR (Basal Metabolic Rate) and the number of calories you are burning throughout the day.

BMR / Basal Metabolic Rate

BMR / Basal Metabolic Rate is essentially the number of calories your body requires while at rest or the minimum number of calories needed for basic vital functions – blood circulation, breathing, etc. Basically, meaning if you did absolutely nothing your body would need x number of calories to survive. There are numerous free online tools to utilize to help in calculating your BMR, which I will let you search online if you prefer. Otherwise, I will introduce a modified version of the Harris-Benedict Formula that will assist with an easy calculation.

- Female = (447.6 + 9.25 x weight in kg) + (3.10 x height in cm) – (4.33 x age in years)
- Male = (88.4 + 13.4 x weight in kg) + (4.8 x height in cm) – 5.68 x age)

To use this formula, you will first need to convert your height and weight into centimeters and kilograms respectively. Let's use an example to illustrate the calculations to clarify using a test subject that is a 40-year-old male who is 5'10 and 175 lbs.

1. Convert height from inches to centimeters – 5 foot 10 inches = 70 inches = **177.8 cm**
2. 1 foot = 12 inches
3. 1 inch = 2.54 centimeters
4. Convert weight from pounds to kilograms – 175 pounds = **79.38 kg**
5. 1 pound = 0.4536 kilograms

Not let's plug in the converted height and weight into the formula to determine the estimated BMR for this test subject.

1. $(447.60 + 9.25 \times \mathbf{79.38}) + (3.10 \times \mathbf{177.80}) - (4.33 \times \mathbf{40})$ = estimated BMR
2. $(1{,}181.87) + (551.18) - (173.20) = \mathbf{1{,}559.85\ calories}$

In this example, the 40-year-old male who is 5'10 at 175 lb has an estimated BMR of about 1,560 calories. I use the term *estimated* as there are many versions of this calculations. This means that he needs approximately 1,560 calories + the number of calories he burns throughout the day to be a net zero, meaning no weight gained and no weight lost. Since we want to be in a caloric surplus to gain size and muscle, we need to ensure what we need increase our calorie intake. This leads to the more difficult part of calculating how many calories you burn throughout the day.

Daily Caloric Expenditure

To get an estimated number of calories burned throughout the day, I suggest purchasing some type of fitness tracker. I won't mention any brand names here but there are many different brands, models, versions, etc. on the market that can vary in price. I suggest doing a quick search to see what fits within your price range to make things a lot easier. And when I say a lot easier, I mean exponentially easier. A version I suggest looking at should also have some type of sleep tracking / monitoring which will be very helpful as adequate rest is vital for maximum recovery.

If obtaining a tracker is not viable, you can find numerous online calculator tools that utilize age, height, weight and activity level. Keep in mind that this should be used as an estimate and illustratively as you incorporate this into your daily routine. It is best to trial and error with your routines for at least a week, preferably a couple weeks to a month and tailor from there depending on your personal results. I ran the test subject above through a couple of online calculators with the average results shown below. Keep in mind that the estimates below will include the BMR calorie count we ran above already.

Estimated Daily Caloric Expenditure Based on Level of Activity:

- Sedentary Lifestyle = 2,052 estimated calories burned
- Light Activity = 2,351 estimated calories burned
- Moderate Activity = 2,651 estimated calories burned
- Very Active = 2,950 estimated calories burned

Why is this important?

This will give you a baseline when anticipating your meal plan that accompanies your new or improved routine. This is a floating and estimated target / range meaning this is not a *calculate once* and use ever day type of thing. You will want to re-assess and calculate along your journey to ensure that you continuously progress. Now that we know approximately how many calories we are burning throughout the day, we can move onto the exciting part of how much calories can we intake. I promise there will be no more brain racking formulas to use here!

Daily Calorie Intake Goal

In general, I would suggest bumping up your calorie intake between 10-20% at first. This will allow you to ease into a caloric surplus without the feeling of discomfort. By increasing your calories by 10-20% you should anticipate around a 0.25% to 0.50% increase in body weight per week, actual results will vary from person to person. Now I know this doesn't sound super appealing at first but remember our goal here – Gain LEAN Muscle. Keeping with our test subject from before, let's use the Very Active lifestyle calorie count above to determine what the target total calorie intake should be.

Very Active Lifestyle = 2.950 calories x 20% increase (to get into a caloric surplus) = 3,540 calories / day

This is great news! Now you can indulge and eat everything in sight! Well, not exactly unless you plan on move into a cutting phase immediately…. To wrap up this section I want to emphasize that the daily calorie count will fluctuate from day to day based on activity level. Sometimes we can get an hour or hour and a half in the gym, some days we can also get in some cardio, some days we are stuck at our desk all day more sedentary, etc. Use your best judgment from day to day to adjust as needed.

Macros

After finding out how many calories we get to intake every day, now it is time to determine where the calories need to come from. When it comes to macros or macro-nutrients, I am referring to protein, carbohydrates and fats. I won't get into the science of how each of the Macros works and reacts with your body in this book as we plan to keep it high level. A gram of protein will not contain the same calorie count as a gram of fats or carbs. To best illustrate this, an estimate that can be used is as follows:

- 1 gram of protein = about 4 calories

- 1 gram of carbs = about 4 calories
- 1 gram of fats = about 9 calories

Also note that the different sources of Macros are not all equal. There are many other factors that come into play. We don't need our science lab coats to tell that a gram of chicken breast is not exactly equivalent to a gram of fried chicken thighs. When considering sources of your Macros, you want to consider as many "clean" sources as possible. This will do a couple of things – allow lean body weight to be added and allow you to eat more since cleaner sources usually carry a lower overall caloric impact. Not to mention keeping you healthy along the way. This isn't to say that you can't indulge on a Saturday night for that slice of birthday cake while at a family party, just make sure to account for it.

I want to address a couple things before I start receiving hate messages as the health industry has many different groups of people with varying degrees of belief that their personal diet or system works better than others. If you are on a Keto Diet, you are vegan or vegetarian, on a paleo diet, a carnivore diet, etc., and it is working for you, that is great. Stick with the nutrition plan that works best for you. What is being shared is a general guideline that has worked for me and a vast majority of fitness enthusiasts in the market. Secondly, this is an absurd simplification. Again, leaving the science lab coats in the closet here, we are not discussing everything in full detail. If you are looking for a deeper dive in the science behind these things, be on the lookout for the longer version and or there is a plethora of research to dig through online. Let's take a deeper dive into the split or ratios of each Macro we should aim to consume, i.e. how many of our daily calories should come from protein, carbs and fats.

Macro Split

When it comes to muscle growth, we want to ensure we are getting an adequate amount of protein as this is the key driver to ensure protein synthesis takes place along with resistance training that breaks down the muscle for it to grow bigger. Carbs are also a very important piece to our plan so we will want to ensure that we are getting adequate levels as well. While in a bulking or gaining phase, you will recall we are in a caloric surplus therefore our bodies are storing the extra calories that we intake which are not burned off. Our bodies store the extra calories that we intake every day in the same form that we intake them, which is why fats and carbs are also an important piece to our plan. But over all we need to intake an adequate level of protein to ensure we capitalize on our gains here, which is why we should focus on forming our nutrition plan around our protein intake.

There is an abundance of research, thoughts, opinions, etc. available online that dives into a macro split. Taking an average and summary of my findings and personal experience, a good rule of thumb is to aim for at least 0.8 to 1 gram of protein per a pound of body weight. This would be a baseline and can be adjusted throughout your program / routine based on your goals and personal results. This would mean that our test subject from our earlier example would need at least 140 to 175 grams of protein. Since the calorie count for protein is around 4 calories per gram of protein, this would provide between 544 to 680 calories. This would be the minimum level of protein to intake during the program for our test subject.

As you recall from our earlier example, our daily calorie intake will vary depending on the level of activity each day. Therefore, an easier approach would be to take your total daily calorie intake and use a ratio of proteins, carbs and fats. We should be using the ratio as a tool to adjust depending on your preference, personal results, etc. Another good rule of thumb is to ensure you get adequate protein and carbs, using the remaining calories for fats. A good ratio to start out with is the following:

- Protein – 20-30% of total calorie intake or around 1+ grams per pound of body weight
- Carbs – 50-60% of total calorie intake or 3+ grams per pound of body weight
- Fats – 20-30% of total calorie intake or the balance of calories that are left

For our test subject from earlier who is 40 years old at 5'10 and 170 lbs, see his macro ratio below for days where he is very active.

- Very Active = 2,950 estimated calories burned
- Protein intake at 20-30% = 590 to 885 calories per day
- Carb intake at 50-60% = 1,475 to 1,770 calories per day
- Fat intake at 20-30% = 590 to 885 calories per day

This would be adjusted depending on his level of activity – sedentary, light, moderate, etc. every day. i.e. he could have a very high caloric need on workout days and a lower caloric count on rest days.

Meal Timing

Now that we have an idea of what our total calorie intake is for the day, let's look at the timing of the meals and how many meals per day to consume all these calories. There are varying thoughts on this which tend to over complicate things. The idea of more frequent small meals throughout the day vs fewer larger meals less frequently vs only consuming calories during a feeding window utilizing some type of fasting, etc. Again, to sound like a broken record, if it is working for you great. Stick with it. I have found my best results by coordinating my meal timing around my workouts. The most important meals of the day will be your pre-workout meal and post workout meal. Reason being you want to ensure that you have enough calories or fuel to power through your workout – pre-workout meal – and enough calories to replenish after the workout – post workout meal. From there you can coordinate a lunch, dinner, before bedtime snack etc. with an even time spacing in between.

For the pre-workout meal it is important to ensure that you account for digestions time. So don't scarf down a huge pre-workout meal and then head straight to the gym. Depending on the type of carbs you intake – complex (whole grains, rice, etc.) vs simple (fruits, sugars, etc.) – you will want to consume your meal around 1-1.5 hours before your workout. As for post workout there is a bit more flexibility. You will want to consume your meal anywhere from 1-3 hours afterwards. So, no need to go speeding off to get your post workout fix. There is also benefits in increasing the level of carb intake pre and post workouts as we are expending a lot of energy. You want to ensure adequate energy to burn pre-workout and replenish post workout.

Now for most of us that are not planning to compete in a body building competition having a dietitian and coach to track all of this for us, although I am sure we could all use this help, a very easy and over simplified way to start out is to take the total number of calories per day and divide by your total number of meals that you plan on eating. As an example, if our test subject from earlier on a very active day is consuming 2,950 calories for the day planning to eat 5 meals per day (pre-workout, post workout, lunch, dinner, pre-bedtime meal), he can aim for around 590 calories per meal.

This is where a macro counting app or online tool will save you a headache. There are many online tools or mobile apps that can help you either calculate calorie counts for whole meals or individual foods. My suggestion is to spend some time on an app or online and research your favorite meals and or regular foods that you eat to get a good idea of their calorie counts. Meal prepping will really help here as you can prepare to ensure that you are in taking exactly what you intend to. It will be eye opening to see what the actual calorie count is for some of your favorite meals. So, as you start your research you are welcome, and I am sorry for bringing this to our attention at the same time.

4

Supplements

When it comes to supplements keep in mind that they are not a requirement, and they are not a sure-fire thing to get you to your goals. They are exactly what they are called – supplements. Meaning they are there to complement and potentially enhance your current routine. Therefore, they are available depending on your comfort level and if you have the resources to obtain them. The supplement market has grown exponentially over the last decade providing a plethora of products within the market. Some of which are amazing and some of which are not so great. Some have a ton of very good research supporting their main functions and some are still in the infancy stages with a lot to be determined regarding their effectiveness, sides affects and efficacy.

Please note that I am not suggesting going out to buy every supplement for what they state they can do by any means. Nor am I suggesting taking supplements at all. This section was intently kept very short and concise for a reason. Future editions will dive into supplements fully. For simplicity, I will limit the number of supplements we discuss focusing on three main supplements – Protein, creatine and a pre-workout supplement.

Protein

As mentioned earlier, protein is a key driver for our goal of gaining lean muscle mass. We want to ensure that we are obtaining not only an adequate level of protein but also elevated levels from what we may be accustomed to normally taking. With these elevated levels it can be difficult to intake fully from whole foods. Therefore, supplementing with protein powder can offer benefits to ensuring we make our target daily macro goals. The suggested use would be as a snack in between meals, part of a pre/post workout meal, taking with a meal to add additional protein or at night as part of your pre-bedtime snack. The benefits of protein supplements include the ease of access since you can pack a shaker literally taking it anywhere with a bottle of water as well as the ability to intake anywhere from 20-50+ grams of protein with a couple swigs.

There are many different types of proteins on the market – concentrate, isolate, casein – as well as many different sources – non-dairy, vegan / plant based, collagen, etc. We will not be diving into the differences and or pros/cons as this topic could be a whole book in itself. The main thing is to look for something within your price range, that sits well with you and tastes great.

Creatine

The second supplement to review is creatine. This is one of the most studied supplements in the market and has been around for decades. Creatine is a non-protein amino acid that can be found in whole foods, generally found in seafood and red meat. Creatine is also an amino acid that the body will naturally produce in small amounts daily. Generally, around a gram per day. This amino acid is stored in your muscles to supplement your energy sources as a key part of energy metabolism.

The suggested benefits of taking creatine include performance Gains – increased capacity for high intensity training, heavier lifting, speed and quickness, etc., recovery – aids with replenishing muscle glycogen levels which can be drained through heavy lifting or high-endurance training, injury prevention – potentially reducing dehydration and much more.

There are many different types of creatines that come in the forms of powders, liquids, pills, etc. that include mono hydrates, hydrochloride, nitrates, etc. Each has different price points, doses, suggested sequencing and so on. Some also suggest a loading phase that will include taking higher doses the first week to fill your "reserves "or bodily "storage". If you are interested in taking creatine, I would suggest spending the time to do some quick research online to determine what will work best for you.

Pre-Workouts

If creatine was confusing, pre-workouts can tend to be just as confusing as well. There is a plethora of options available when it comes to the "pre-workout" category. Pre-workout supplements are generally taking around 30 minutes before your workout to provide a bit of a boost in energy and enhanced performance with an increase in blood flow. Depending on the source, the supplement can contain different vitamins, nutrients, stimulants, etc. This can be as simple as a cup of coffee or as complex as series of supplements. Again, use your judgment on what works best for you.

If you choose to utilize a pre-workout supplement, please proceed with caution as some of the products in the market contain a very high level of stimulants (generally in the form of caffeine). So, when starting with a new product, I always suggest checking the label to ensure you are aware of what the potential impacts can be. It doesn't hurt to start off with half of the suggested dose to see how you react as well.

When considering a pre-workout product, I have found the best results with products that contain a blend of Amino Acids, Beta-alanine, creatine, a low level of glucose, nitric oxide and a blend of vitamins. I won't mention any brand names and or dive into each of the ingredients above in full detail. But the general a pre-workout should help with providing a boost of energy – allowing you to train harder or longer or both without risk of injury, increased blood flow – increasing the flow of blood to your muscles and improved recovery aiding with growth and repair.

5

Work Out Splits

With our newly established foundational knowledge of a developing a muscle building program we are ready to dive into a couple different workout splits or training routines. We will look at four specific workout splits as an introduction which can be adjusted and or rotated depending on your personal preference, time availability, access to equipment, etc. The four splits are a Full Body, Upper/Lower, Push Pull Legs (PPL) and a Classic Split (commonly referred to as a "Bro" split). Each split has endless variations as you rotate specific exercises. Each workout will also likely include a combination of both compound and isolation exercises. A compound exercise includes movements that activate multiple muscle groups together such as dead lifts, squats, bench press, etc. An isolation exercise includes movements that are specifically concentrated on a particular muscle such as preacher bicep curl, cable triceps kickback, lateral cable raise, etc. By using a combination of compound and isolation movements we can maximize our growth potential. With that said, let's look at the suggested workout splits a bit more. Keep in mind that to get an adequate quick warm up in including stretching, light cardio, foam rolling, etc. before each workout session as well as a couple of warm up sets before starting your working set. Let's jump in.

Full Body

A full body split is exactly what it sounds like, a full body workout whereas you will work a large majority of your muscle groups every workout. These workouts usually include mostly compound movements such as squats, bench press, overhead press, etc. The benefit of this type of workout split is that you will maximize your time in the gym by hitting a large group of muscles as well as a high caloric burn from the compound movements. For this workout split it will be important to ensure you get an adequate amount of rest allowing your muscles to recover and grow. This split can be beneficial if you do not have multiple days or time to commit to working out. The downfalls of this workout split are that you will not get very much volume per each muscle group, unless you work out more than twice per week. This is a good intermediate to advance workout split. A couple examples of weekly workout routines can include the following:

Sample # 1
   Monday – Full Body Workout #1
   Tuesday – Rest
   Wednesday – Full Body Workout #2
   Thursday – Rest
   Friday – Full Body Workout #3
   Saturday – Rest
   Sunday – Rest

Sample # 2
   Monday – Full Body Workout #1
   Tuesday – Rest

Wednesday – Rest

Thursday – Full Body Workout #2

Friday – Rest

Saturday – Rest

Sunday – Rest

Full Body Workout # 1

Exercise	Rep Range	# of Sets
Barbell Squat	8-10	4
Dumbbell Single Arm Row	8-10	4
Dumbbell Bench Press	8-10	4
Walking Lunge with Dumbbells	10	4
Incline Seated Dumbbell Curl	10-12	3
Standing Overhead Triceps Extension with Bar	10-12	3
Calf Raise Machine	10-12	3
Cable Crunch	12-15	3

Full Body Workout # 2

Exercise	Rep Range	# of Sets
Barbell Bench Press	8-10	4
Cable / Machine Fly	10-12	3
Machine Leg Extension	8-10	4
Machine Lying Leg Curl	8-10	4
Pull Up (weighted or with body weight)	8-10	4
Cable Lateral Raise	8-10	4
Preacher Dumbbell Hammer Curl	10-12	3
Cable Rope Pull Downs	10-12	3
Cable Crunch	12-15	3

Full Body Workout #3

Exercise	Rep Range	# of Sets
Barbell Deadlift	8-10	4
Seated Dumbbell Press	8-10	4
Barbell Front Raise	8-10	4
Wide Grip Lat Pull Down	8-10	4
Machine Leg Press	8-10	4
Barbell Curl (EZ Bar)	8-10	3
Seated Dumbbell Skull Crusher	8-10	3
Machine Shrugs	8-10	3
Cable Crunch	8-10	3

Upper / Lower

The upper / lower workout split is similar to the full body workout split but breaks out the upper and lower body movements into different days. This will allow you to still hit multiple muscle groups each day while providing a bit more volume per each muscle group which will help with continued gains. This workout split usually consists of compound movements as well which will also tend to generate a higher caloric burn potentially generating a good amount of fat loss also. Since you are hitting multiple muscle groups with a bit more volume and more frequency there should be an ample amount of rest to ensure continued gains. This is a good intermediate to advance workout split. A couple of sample weekly schedules may include the following.

Sample # 1
   Monday – Upper Body #1
   Tuesday – Lower Body #1
   Wednesday – Rest
   Thursday – Upper Body #2
   Friday – Lower Body #2
   Saturday – Rest
   Sunday – Rest

Sample # 2
   Monday – Upper Body #1
   Tuesday – Lower Body #1
   Wednesday – Rest
   Thursday – Rest
   Friday – Upper Body #2
   Saturday – Lower Body #2
   Sunday – Rest

Upper Body Workout #1

Exercise	Rep Range	# of Sets
Barbell Bench Press	8-10	4
Wide Grip Lat Pull Down	10-12	4
Incline Dumbbell Press	10-12	4
Seated Cable Row (close grip)	10-12	4
Dumbbell Shoulder Press	8-10	4
Incline Dumbbell Curl	10-12	3
Triceps Press Down with Rope	10-12	3

Lower Body Workout #1

Exercise	Rep Range	# of Sets
Barbell Squat	8	4
Roman Barbell Deadlift	10-12	4
Machine Leg Extension	10-12	4
Seated Machine Leg Curl	10-12	4
Standing Machine Calf Raise	10-12	4

Upper Body Workout #2

Exercise	Rep Range	# of Sets
Incline Barbell Bench Press	10-12	4
Reverse Grip Lat Pull Down with Bar	10-12	4
Cable Flys (neutral)	10-12	4
Bent Over Barbell Row	8-10	4
Lateral Dumbbell Raise	10-12	3
EZ Bar Preacher Curl	10-12	3
Lying Dumbbell Pull Overs	10-12	3

Lower Body Workout #2

Exercise	Rep Range	# of Sets
Barbell Deadlift	8-10	4
Machine Leg Press	8-10	4
Dumbbell Bulgarian Split Squat	8-10	4
Machine Lying Leg Curl	10-12	3
Seated Calf Raise Machine	10-12	3

Push, Pull, Legs (PPL)

A push, pull, legs workout split is similar to a full body workout and upper / lower body workout in the sense that you are working multiple muscle groups every workout, but you will be focusing on the type of movement specific to the pushing and pulling movements for the upper body separate from the lower body. In my opinion this is an ideal workout split which will provide the benefits of both splits previously mentioned while maximizing workload / volume along with a high caloric burn. This should help in achieving our main goal here – adding lean muscle mass. One potential downfall to this workout split is that multiple days are needed, and the cycle may not perfectly align with a calendar week. Therefore, I would recommend this spit as more advanced taking into account the time dedication and tracking for this routine. A sample weekly schedule may include the following:

Sample # 1
   Monday – Push Workout #1
   Tuesday – Pull Workout #1
   Wednesday – Legs Workout #1
   Thursday – Rest
   Friday – Push Workout #2
   Saturday – Pull Workout #2
   Sunday – Legs Workout #2

Sample # 2
   Monday – Push Workout #1
   Tuesday – Pull Workout #1
   Wednesday – Legs Workout #1
   Thursday – Push Workout #2
   Friday – Pull Workout #2
   Saturday – Legs Workout #2
   Sunday – Rest

Push Workout #1

Exercise	Rep Range	# of Sets
Dumbbell Bench Press	8-10	4
Incline Barbell Bench Press	8-10	4
Cable Flys	10-12	3
Seated Dumbbell Shoulder Press	8-10	4
Dumbbell Front Raise	8-10	3
Cable Lateral Raise	10-12	3
Lying Barbell Triceps Extension	10-12	3
Cable Triceps Press Down with Bar	10-12	3

Pull Workout #1

Exercise	Rep Range	# of Sets
Barbell Deadlift	8-10	4
Wide Grip Lat Pull Down	8-10	4
Barbell Row	8-10	4
Single Arm Dumbbell Row	10-12	3
Reverse Cable Flys	10-12	3
Barbell Curl (narrow grip)	8-10	4
Incline Dumbbell Curl	8-10	3
Pull Up	AMRAP*	3
*AMRAP = as many as possible		

Legs Workout #1

Exercise	Rep Range	# of Sets
Machine Leg Extensions	8-10	4
Machine Leg Press	8-10	4
Reverse Dumbbell Lunges	10-12	4
Roman Deadlift	8-10	4
Machine Leg Curl	10-12	4
Standing Calf Raise	10-12	4

Push Workout #2

Exercise	Rep Range	# of Sets
Barbell Bench Press	8-10	4
Incline Dumbbell Bench Press	8-10	4
Dips (weighted or non-weighted)	10-12	4
Seated Barbell Military Press	8-10	4
Dumbbell Lateral Raise	10-12	3
Close-Grip Barbell Bench Press	10-12	3
Overhead Cable Rope Extensions	10-12	4

Pull Workout #2

Exercise	Rep Range	# of Sets
Reverse Grip Lat Pull Down	8-10	4
Seated Cable Row (close grip)	8-10	4
Chest Supported Dumbbell Row	10-12	4
Dumbbell Shrug	8-10	3
Back Extension (weighted or non-weighted)	10-12	3
Dumbbell Hammer Preacher Curl	10-12	3
Seated Barbell Curl (EZ Bar / wide grip)	8-10	3

Legs Workout #2

Exercise	Rep Range	# of Sets
Barbell Squat	8-10	5
Machine Leg Press	8-10	4
Machine Leg Extension	10-12	4
Seated Leg Curl	10-12	4

Classic / "Bro" Split

The last workout split to mention here is the classic / "bro" split which will break out each muscle group into separate days. This will allow the maximum amount of volume (since each day is dedicated to a specific muscle group) and rest as you will likely only be working each muscle group primarily once per a week or cycle. Keep in mind multiple muscle groups will be engaged each day but will only be the primary emphasis one day per week. This routine would be in the category of intermediate to advanced since there is a high dedication of time and volume associated. There will tend to be more soreness with this split as well since you will be focusing on one muscle group primarily each day. A couple of samples for this weekly cycle can be as follows:

Sample # 1

    Monday – Chest / Triceps Workout

    Tuesday – Back / Bicep Workout

    Wednesday – Rest

    Thursday – Shoulders Workout

    Friday – Legs Workout

Saturday – Rest

Sunday – Rest

Sample # 2

Monday – Chest Workout

Tuesday – Back / Bicep Workout

Wednesday – Shoulder Workout

Thursday – Legs Workout

Friday – Bicep / Triceps Workout

Saturday – Rest

Sunday – Rest

Chest / Triceps Work Out

Exercise	Rep Range	# of Sets
Barbell Incline Bench Press	8-10	4
Dumbbell Bench Press	8-10	4
Decline Dumbbell Bench Press	8-10	4
Cable Flys (high and low)	10-12	3
Cable Triceps Rope Pull Down	10-12	4
Dips	10-12	3

Back / Biceps Work Out

Exercise	Rep Range	# of Sets
Wide Grip Lat Pull Down	8-10	4
Barbell Deadlift	8-10	4
Bent Over Barbell Row	8-10	3
Singe Arm Dumbbell Row	10-12	3
Reverse Cable Flye	10-12	3
Preacher Barbell Curl	8-10	4
Incline Dumbbell Curl	10-12	3

Shoulder Workout

Exercise	Rep Range	# of Sets
Barbell Military Press	8-10	4
Dumbbell Lateral Raise	8-10	4
Dumbbell Front Raise	8-10	4
Bent Over Reverse Dumbbell Flys	10-12	3
Dumbbell Shrugs	8-10	3

Legs Workout

Exercise	Rep Range	# of Sets
Barbell Squats	8-10	4
Roman Barbell Deadlifts	8-10	4
Dumbbell Walking Lunges	10-12	3
Machine Leg Extensions	10-12	3
Lying Leg Curls	10-12	3
Standing Calf Raise	10-12	3

Alternative Arm Work Out (if arms trained separate)

Exercise	Rep Range	# of Sets
Barbell Preacher Curl	8-10	4
Lying Barbell Triceps Extension	8-10	4
Incline Dumbbell Curl	10-12	3
Cable Rope Pull Down	10-12	3
Dumbbell Hammer Curl	10-12	3
Overhead Cable Triceps Extension	10-12	3

6

Conclusion

If you made it this far, congrats! You should now have a good foundational knowledge of what it will take to setup a lean muscle building routine. My hope here was to provide a baseline starting point for everyone to use moving forward immediately as well as in the future along your fitness journey as you continue to evolve along the way. Keep in mind that this is an introductory book that is only scratching the surface. As our routines develop and become more complex, each of the topics discussed can be further explored in much more detail and I hope you continue learning more about each topic. I have enjoyed being your guide and look forward to continuing to do so in future editions.

If you found this book to be helpful in anyway, I would be very grateful and appreciative if you left a favorable review for the book in Amazon. This will help me continue to grow as well.

Resources

Krzysztofik, N., Wilk, N., Wojdała, N., & Gołaś, N. (2019). Maximizing Muscle Hypertrophy: A Systematic review of advanced resistance training techniques and methods. *International Journal of Environmental Research and Public Health/International Journal of Environmental Research and Public Health, 16*(24), 4897. https://doi.org/10.3390/ijerph162448 97

Frothingham, S. (2024, June 11). *Hypertrophy Training vs. Strength Training: Pros and Cons.* Healthline. https://www.healthline.com/hea lth/exercise-fitness/hypertrophy-vs-strength#hypertrophy-vs-streng th

Cssd, E. S. R. (2023, May 8). How to Build Muscle: What to Eat, How to Train & Everything in Between. *Trifecta.* https://www.trifectanutrit ion.com/blog/how-to-gain-muscle-mass-the-ultimate-guide

Cpt, P. W. (2021, May 20). *How to calculate your basal metabolic Rate (BMR).* Verywell Fit. https://www.verywellfit.com/basal-metabolic-rate-1229751

Cscs, D. P. R. (2020, October 8). *Clean Bulking: Overview, guide, and best foods.* Healthline. https://www.healthline.com/nutrition/clean-bulk#

steps

St Pierre Ms Rd, B. (2023, December 10). *How to count (and track) macros for fat loss, muscle gain, and better health.* Precision Nutrition. https://www.precisionnutrition.com/how-to-count-macros

Deldicque, L. (2020). Protein intake and Exercise-Induced Skeletal Muscle Hypertrophy: An update. *Nutrients, 12*(7), 2023. https://doi.org/10.3390/nu12072023

Witard, O. C., Bannock, L., & Tipton, K. D. (2022). Making sense of muscle protein synthesis: A focus on muscle growth during resistance training. *International Journal of Sport Nutrition and Exercise Metabolism, 32*(1), 49–61. https://doi.org/10.1123/ijsnem.2021-0139

Pts, S. D. a. M. W. B. (2024, February 7). *The best macros for bulking: How much protein, carbs & fat to eat.* Bony to Beastly. https://bonytobeastly.com/bulking-macros/

Set, S. F. (2024, June 7). *The difference between concentric and eccentric muscle contraction.* SET FOR SET. https://www.setforset.com/blogs/news/concentric-vs-eccentric-muscle-contraction

Creatine. (2023, December 13). Mayo Clinic. https://www.mayoclinic.org/drugs-supplements-creatine/art-20347591